Apple Cider Vinegar

100+ Tips and Tricks for Healthy Home and Healthy Body

Joanne Hillyer

CONTENTS

INTRODUCTION

Thank you for taking the time to download this book: *Apple Cider Vinegar: 100+ Tips and Tricks for Healthy Home and Healthy Body.*

My passion is health and wellness, especially forms and methods that are alternative to traditional/pharmaceutical medicine. This book covers the topic of Apple Cider Vinegar (ACV), and its many benefits as a cheap and easy household remedy.

By the end of this book you will have a good understanding of what ACV is and the many, many uses for it in cooking, cleaning, body care, first aid, beauty, and health.

Once again, thank you for your purchase of this book, I hope you find it to be helpful!

1 WHAT IS APPLE CIDER VINEGAR?

Apple cider vinegar (ACV) is a type of vinegar that is made from apple must (juice) or cider, the alcoholic beverage made from fermented apple juice. It usually appears pale to medium amber in color.

ACV is commonly used in salad dressings, vinaigrettes, marinades, food preservatives, and chutneys. It is produced by crushing and squeezing apples. Yeast and bacteria are added to the liquid to begin its alcoholic fermentation process when the sugars are converted to alcohol. A second fermentation process takes place to convert alcohol to vinegar by the acetic acid-forming bacteria, known as acetobacter. The malic acid and acetic acid created from the fermentation processes give vinegar its distinct sour taste.

ACV is the most popular type of vinegar. Vinegar has been used for a variety of household and cooking purposes for centuries. There are also claims of its excellent medicinal benefits.

Benefits of Apple Cider Vinegar

ACV has countless benefits for body care, beauty, cleaning, and first aid. Among the many uses you will learn about in the next chapters, ACV …

- Detoxifies the home. Because it is made from fermented apple juice, you can use it to replace other housecleaning products, thereby immediately decreasing your consumption of unnatural and harmful chemicals in your home and daily life.

- Can be used to care for your hair. You can use apple cider vinegar for rinsing after washing your hair. It gives your hair natural shine and body. To use it, fill an empty shampoo bottle with 1 cup cold water and ½ tablespoon apple cider vinegar. Simply rinse your hair with the solution after shampooing. It is safe for use several times a week.

1

- Helps regulate the natural pH level of the skin

- Can be used as a toner

- Removes stains from your teeth

- Can help soothe sunburns

- Aids in weight loss

- Helps maintain the balance in the functions of the body's inner system

- Can be used as a detoxifying agent

- Helps cleanse your lymph nodes by helping break down mucus, thereby helping in sinus decongestion

- The natural enzymes in apple cider vinegar help in the treatment of candida infection

- Aids in reducing heartburn

- Known to lower bad cholesterol levels

- An excellent antioxidant

- Helps in regulating blood sugar levels

- Can be used as a laxative

- Helps repeal fleas from your pets

- Acts as a natural room freshener

- Can be used as a natural deodorant

- Helps ease the symptoms of the common cold

- Removes warts

- Makes a good acid efflux treatment

- Has anti-fungal properties

- Helps heal poison ivy

- Helps fight allergies

- Helps ease varicose veins

- Can be used for household cleaning chores

Why is ACV Good for You?

Apple cider vinegar contains many nutrients that your body needs: essential vitamins, minerals, organic acids, amino acids, and polyphenolic compounds (micronutrients that help prevent diseases). ACV also contains pectin, which is an insoluble fiber that can be found in fruits and plants. Pectin is rich in fiber, so your body can benefit greatly from consistently including ACV in your daily regimen. It is a good prebiotic, which supports the growth of probiotic bacteria and promotes a healthy gut.

These are just some of the most notable benefits of increasing your intake of ACV daily. The coming chapters you cover practical applications for the use of ACV.

2 APPLE CIDER VINEGAR FOR COOKING

Apple cider vinegar has been used for centuries. ACV is so versatile that you can use it for cooking, cleaning, caring for the skin, and for maintaining your overall well-being, among other uses.

There are countless ways that you can incorporate apple cider vinegar into your regular routine. One of the most important uses for ACV is for cooking. In this chapter, you'll find helpful tips and some recipes that you can easily follow.

Use it as a salad dressing

Apple cider vinegar is a good replacement for balsamic vinegar when making your own salad dressing.

Honey Vinaigrette Dressing

Ingredients

- ¼ cup apple cider vinegar
- ¾ cup olive oil
- 2 tbsp. honey
- 2 tbsp. water
- ¼ tsp ground pepper
- 1 ½ tsp salt

Salad Toppings

Your choice of:

- Apples
- Spinach
- Raisins
- Walnuts

The toppings will depend on what you prefer or what is available in your pantry. Dare to experiment until you arrive at the perfect combination.

How to Prepare

- In a blender, mix vinegar, water, salt, honey, salt, and pepper.
- Gradually add olive oil into the blender, making sure that it yields a smooth consistency.
- Toss the dressing into your vegetable salad.
- Enjoy.

Add it to a smoothie

You can add a few drops when you drink your morning smoothie to provide you with more energy.

Use it when cooking rice

Add a few drops to rice water when cooking rice. It will give you fluffier cooked rice.

Use it as a replacement for white vinegar

Apple cider vinegar is a healthier alternative for your regular white vinegar for your cooking needs.

Wash fruits and vegetables with it

You can add apple cider vinegar to the water you will use to wash your fruits and vegetables.

Add it to your beverages

You can make a healthy tonic with apple cider vinegar. Simply combine apple cider vinegar, distilled water, honey, and organic cayenne pepper.

Make your tomato juice healthier by adding a shot of apple cider vinegar.

Here's an easy recipe for a good thirst quencher:

ACV Tonic

- Combine 1 to 2 tbsps. of apple cider vinegar with 8 oz. of purified water.
- You may opt to add 1 to 2 tsps. organic honey.
- You can add in a few drops of liquid stevia.
- For added sweetness, add in 1 to 2 tsp. maple syrup.

Apple cider vinegar is versatile enough that you can add it to your favorite fruit or vegetable juice, smoothie, or shake.

Add it to stews and soups

Apple cider vinegar makes a good addition to stews and soups to enhance the flavor. Adding just a few drops when the stew or soup is nearly done cooking can make a huge difference in the taste.

Replace salt with it

If your diet calls for reducing your consumption of salt and sodium, you can use apple cider vinegar as an alternative. You can sprinkle a few drops of ACV on rice, raw vegetables, and nearly any dish to bring out the amazing flavors of your favorite ingredients.

Add it to sauces

Apple cider vinegar has a tangy and fruity taste that can be used to enhance the flavor of your favorite sauce. It helps soften vegetables faster when you add ACV while cooking. Add ACV when cooking with tomato sauce. It makes a good complement because both these ingredients are acidic.

Use it when boiling eggs

Try adding a tablespoon of apple cider vinegar when boiling eggs. It helps prevent the shells from cracking while boiling, thus preventing the whites from leaking out.

Use it in a marinade

When you use apple cider vinegar to marinate meat, it helps tenderize the protein and kills any bacteria. In a mixing bowl, mix ¾-cup apple cider vinegar and the herbs and spices you will be using for the marinade. Let the meat rest in this mixture for a few hours. You'll get even better results when you leave it overnight. Grill the protein as you usually would and enjoy.

Use it as a food preservative

ACV is a good preservative, so you can add it to any food you wish to keep and enjoy over the next few days.

Extend the freshness of fruits

Soak fruits (even vegetables) for a few minutes in a mixture of 7/8th water to 1/8th apple cider vinegar. It will help prevent the fruits you've already sliced from turning brown. To retain the vibrant color of your vegetables try adding 1 tbsp. of cider vinegar while boiling them.

As a substitute for many things

Apple cider vinegar is a good substitute for any acidic ingredient such as lemon. When mixed with garlic and pepper you get an added tangy flavor to your dish. You also can substitute eggs with apple cider vinegar when baking at a ratio of 1 tbsp. of ACV for each egg used.

As an addition to your favorite soup recipe

Apple cider vinegar can enhance the flavor of this low-calorie chicken soup recipe:

Low-Calorie Chicken Soup

Ingredients

- 1 pound chicken breast
- 2 ½ tbsp. olive oil
- 4 cloves of garlic (diced)
- 1 medium onion (chopped)
- 3 stalks of celery (chopped)
- 3 cups kale (chopped)
- 1 pound sweet potatoes (peeled and chopped)
- 10 grape tomatoes (cut in halves)
- 2 tbsp. apple cider vinegar
- 3 cups of water
- 3 cups chicken broth
- Sea salt
- Ground pepper
- Fresh ginger (optional)

How to Prepare

- Season the chicken breasts with sea salt and pepper.
- Heat a soup pot over medium-high heat.
- Put olive oil and cook chicken until golden brown on each side (about 4 minutes per side).
- Remove chicken from heat and set aside.
- On the same pot, add celery, onion, and garlic.

- Cook until tender.

- Add in apple cider vinegar, and then add sweet potatoes, tomatoes, kale, water, and chicken broth.

- Bring to a boil.

- Reduce heat and simmer for about 20 minutes.

- While soup is cooking, shred chicken (using your hands), then add into the pot.

- Simmer for another 2 to 3 minutes.

- Serve hot with grated fresh ginger (optional).

Tenderize meat

To tenderize meat, add 1 tablespoon of ACV per quarter pound of meat roughly 15 minutes before cooking.

Add flavor to recipes

Simple Chicken Dish

<u>Ingredients</u>

- 1 pound sweet potatoes (cut into chunks)
- 2 medium-sized apples (cored, cut into chunks, unpeeled)
- 1 tbsp. fresh ginger (chopped)
- 1 cup apple cider vinegar
- ½ tsp. cinnamon
- Dried apple chips (optional)

<u>How to Prepare</u>

- In a large cooking pot, mix together all ingredients, except for the dried apple chips.
- Bring to a boil.
- Reduce heat and cover pot. Simmer for 30 minutes.
- Let it cool down before pureeing until smooth in a blender. Do it by batch.
- Serve topped with dried apple chips.

Enhance the flavor of bone broth

Bone broth has now become popular because it makes a healthy and delicious soup. Take two cups of this every morning and you have all the energy you need for the whole day. It is also a great source of hydration. It also benefits people suffering from insomnia as it helps you sleep soundly at night.

Bone Broth

Ingredients

- 2 lbs. beef bones
- 3 carrots (cut in half)
- 3 stalks of celery (halved)
- 1 medium-sized onion (halved)
- ¼ cup apple cider vinegar
- 12 cups water

How to Prepare

- Put all the ingredients in a slow cooker.
- Set to low heat.
- Cook for 15 hours.
- Let it cool, and then strain it.
- Transfer the strained broth into mason jars.
- Skim fat off the top.
- Put in the refrigerator or freezer.
- Take out one Mason jar when you're ready to drink it. Skim off remaining fat and reheat.
- This recipe makes approximately 12 cups.

Enhance the flavor of your favorite salad

This is an easy to make salad that you can create in minutes. You can even prepare ·
it beforehand for a quick office lunch. This is high in fiber and rich in protein, as it
also contains black beans. Avocados are rich in omega-3s, essential vitamins, and
minerals.

Avocado Black Bean Salad

Ingredients

- 2 cups avocados (diced)
- 4 cups black beans (cooked)
- 2 cups onions (diced)
- 2 tbsp. flaxseed oil (or olive oil or vegetable oil)
- 2 tsp. maple syrup (or you can use honey)
- 3 tbsp. apple cider vinegar
- Salt

How to Prepare

- In a mixing bowl, combine black beans, avocados, and onion.
- Whisk together oil, maple syrup (or honey), apple cider vinegar, and a
  pinch of salt, in another bowl.
- Toss and serve.

3 RECIPES THAT USE APPLE CIDER VINEGAR

Apple cider vinegar is great for cooking because of its versatility. It's more than just your regular vinegar. This chapter is dedicated to a variety of recipes that you can easily follow and do at home.

Grilled Halibut with Vinaigrette

Serve this when you have your in-laws over and they'll love you for it.

Ingredients

- 2 halibut fillets (roughly 4 ounces each)
- 1 large gold beet (peeled, boiled, diced)
- 1 large beet (peeled, boiled, diced)
- ¼ cup farro
- 1 crisp apple (diced)
- 2 tbsp. extra-virgin olive oil
- 1 tbsp. apple cider vinegar
- 2 tbsp. pistachios (chopped)
- 2 scallions (sliced)
- Salt & pepper

How to Prepare

- Season halibut with salt and pepper. Brush with oil. Set aside.

- In a large saucepan, boil 2 quarts salted water and cook beets until tender (approximately 30 to 40 minutes). Allow the beets to cool down at room temperature before you peel and slice them.

- In a saucepan, cook farro with 1 cup salted water, simmer until tender or until water has been absorbed (approximately 20 minutes).

- In a large salad bowl, whisk ACV, olive oil, scallions, and pistachios. Add beets, farro, and apples. Toss gently. Set aside.

- Grill halibut fillet over medium to high heat (roughly 5 minutes on each side).

- Divide the farro salad into 2 plates and top with a piece of grilled halibut. Garnish with sliced scallions.

Brussels Sprouts Slaw with a Twist

Ingredients

- 2 pounds Brussels sprouts (sliced thinly with a food processor)
- ¾ pound thick-cut bacon (chopped into half inch pieces)
- 2 green apples (peeled, coarsely grated, squeezed dry)
- 4 tbsp. unsalted butter
- 1 tsp fresh thyme leave
- 1 tsp. fresh ginger (minced)
- 1 tbsp. apple cider vinegar
- 1 pinch of salt
- Freshly ground black pepper

How to Prepare

- In a skillet, cook bacon until crisp, over medium to high heat. Drain excess oil. Save the bacon fat for later.
- Turn the heat up to high, on the same skillet, add 2 tbsps. of butter and 2 tbsps. of bacon fat.
- Add half of the Brussels sprouts. Cook until soft, stirring often.
- Add salt and pepper to taste. Remove and set aside. Cook the remaining Brussels sprouts in the remaining 2 tbsps. butter and 2 tsps. bacon fat.
- Add the first batch of cooked sprouts. And then add the apples, ginger, thyme, and ACV. Stir until the apples are heated, roughly 1 to 2 minutes.
- Arrange the slaw on a platter. Top with cooked bacon before serving.

Garden Salad with Salmon

Try using salmon in your salad instead of chicken. It's healthy as salmon is rich in omega-3 fatty acids and other essential vitamins.

Ingredients

- 1 cup canned salmon (coarsely chopped)
- 1 cup fennel bulb (diced)
- 1 cup cucumber (diced)
- 1 cup red onions (diced)
- 2 tbsps. olive oil
- 3 tbsps. apple cider vinegar

How to Prepare

- Combine all ingredients in a large salad bowl.
- Gently toss and serve.

Not Your Ordinary Deviled Egg

Here's a different take on a classic.

Ingredients

- 6 eggs
- 1 cup apple cider vinegar
- 1 can/jar pickled beets (16-oz)
- 1 tsp. Dijon mustard
- 1/3 cup brown sugar
- 1 tbsp. mayonnaise
- 1 tsp. salt
- 1 tbsp. peppercorns
- ½ tsp. curry powder
- 2 tbsps. olive oil
- 1 tbsp. vinegar
- Salt & ground pepper
- Fresh rosemary (chopped)

How to Prepare

- Hard boil the eggs and peel off shells. Set aside.
- *How to make the brine*:

   In a bowl or jar, put the pickled beets.

   Add apple cider vinegar, peppercorns, salt, and sugar.

   Stir well.

- Add the eggs to the brine. Cover and place in the refrigerator for about 12 hours. You may keep the eggs in the brine for up to 3 days. Keeping the eggs longer in the brine will give you a sourer and pinker (in color). Ideally, 16 hours in the refrigerator would get good results.

- Slice the eggs in half. Scoop out all the yolks and place in another bowl. Add mustard, curry, mayonnaise, olive oil, and vinegar into the yolks. Mix well and mash until you get a smooth consistency. Add a water if the mixture becomes too stiff. Add salt and ground pepper for flavor.

- With a pastry bag (alternative: regular plastic bag), pipe off the yolk mixture into the hollow in each of the eggs.

- Garnish with rosemary on top.

Cabbage Salad with Vinaigrette

This recipe would make a good side dish to your favorite steak or other meat dish.

Ingredients

- 5 cups red cabbage (thinly sliced)

- 4 oz. lettuce (sliced into strips or torn)

- 2 medium-sized carrots (sliced into ribbons, using a vegetable peeler)

- 2 medium-sized apples, use the crisp variety, like Gala, Sweet Tango, (diced)

- 2 cauliflower (finely chopped)

- ½ cup scallions (thinly sliced)

- 1 ½ tbsps. mayonnaise

- 3 tbsps. canola oil (you can also use safflower, vegetable, or mild nut oil)

- ½ tsp. brown sugar

- 3 tbsps. apple cider vinegar

- ¼ tsp. Dijon mustard

- 5 grinds freshly ground pepper

- A pinch of sea salt

- ½ cup toasted pepitas

How to Prepare

- In a large salad (mixing) bowl, mix together lettuce, cabbage, carrots, cauliflower, apples, and scallions. Toss until the carrots are tangled with the cabbage shreds and lettuce leaves, and the apples and cauliflower settle throughout, instead of getting stuck at the bottom of the bowl.

- In a different bowl, whisk mayonnaise and oil until smooth. Add mustard and sugar, and whisk again. Lastly, add in vinegar, salt, and pepper until it emulsifies into a dressing.

- Pour the vinaigrette over your beets salad, top with pepitas, and toss again.

- Serve immediately.

Not Your Regular Waldorf Salad

The usual Waldorf salad has apples, walnuts, and celery with mayonnaise as dressing. This one has apples and chicken, and yogurt, enhanced with apple cider vinegar.

Ingredients

½ cup plain yogurt

1 tsp. Dijon mustard

2 tbsps. apple cider vinegar

1 tsp. honey

½ tsp. sea salt

12 tsp. red pepper flakes (crushed)

¼ tsp. freshly ground black pepper

1 can chickpeas (14-ounce variety, drained and rinsed)

2 ribs celery (finely chopped)

1 medium-sized apples (chunks)

¼ cup parsley (chopped)

½ cup walnuts (chopped)

4 cups fresh spinach

How to Prepare

- Prepare the dressing by combining yogurt, mustard, honey, salt, pepper flakes, pepper, and apple cider vinegar in a mixing bowl. Whisk until completely mixed.

- In a large salad bowl, put in apples, grapes, celery, onions, walnuts, and parsley.

- Pour in the dressing and toss well.

- Refrigerate for at least 30 minutes before serving.

- This can last up to 5 days in the refrigerator.

JOANNE HILLYER

Switchel

You must try this unique drink for this summer. It's a refreshing new take on an old-fashioned drink, the switchel.

Ingredients

- 2 tbsps. apple cider vinegar

- 4 tbsps. sweetener (maple syrup, sugar, honey, molasses)

- ¼ tsp. ground ginger or 1 tsp. fresh ginger (grated)

- 1 cup water

How to Prepare

- Mix everything in a medium-sized glass or Mason jar.

- Cover and put in the refrigerator for at least 2 hours or up to 24 hours.

- Shake or stir well before serving the drink.

- You can adjust the taste to your preference.

- If you opt to use fresh ginger, strain through a fine cheesecloth.

- Serve with ice or mix with soda water, if you want.

Delicious Sardine Toast

This is a new take on your favorite snack or breakfast, the toast.

Ingredients

Pickled Onions:

- 1 red onion (small, thinly sliced)
- ½ cup water
- ½ tsp. granulated sugar
- ½ tsp. fine salt
- ½ cup apple cider vinegar

Toast

- 4 pieces crisp bread or crackers
- 1 can sardines (3.5 oz.)
- 4 tsps. Dijon mustard

How to Prepare

- *For the pickled onions:* In a saucepan over medium to high heat, bring to a boil water, apple cider vinegar, sugar, and salt, stirring occasionally to dissolve sugar and salt. Remove from heat, and then add onions. Let it stand for 15 minutes. Store in an airtight container and place in the refrigerator. It can be stored for up to a month.

- *For the toasts:* Spread 1 tsp. of mustard on each piece of crisp bread. Distribute the sardines among the crisp breads. Gently smash into bread with a fork. Add a thin layer of pickled onions.

- Serve immediately.

- *Note:* You can use either oil-based or water-based sardines.

Vegan Cheesy Dip

Ingredients

- 2 tbsps. olive oil
- ½ large yellow onion (diced)
- 3 cloves garlic (pressed)
- 2 large carrots (finely chopped)
- 1 cup butternut squash (thinly sliced)
- 2 tsps. salt (divided)
- 1 tsp. cumin
- ¼ tsp. black pepper
- ½ tsp. chili powder
- 1 can green chilies
- 1 cup vegetable stock
- 1 cup cashew nuts (soaked for at least 30 minutes to overnight, drained)
- 1 ½ cups plain, unsweetened almond milk
- ½ cup salsa
- ¼ cup nutritional yeast
- 1 tbsp. apple cider vinegar
- *Other possible toppings:* chopped cherry tomatoes, pickled jalapenos, cilantro

How to Prepare

- Heat saucepan over medium-high heat, add olive oil. Once hot, sauté garlic and onions until soft and fragrant.
- Add carrots and butternut squash.

- Add 1 tsp. salt, chili powder, cumin, and black pepper. Cook for another couple of minutes, and then add the vegetable stock.

- Let it simmer, stirring often, until vegetables are cooked.

- Put the vegetables into a high-powered blender. Add chilies, cashew nuts, almond milk, yeast, apple cider vinegar, salsa, and the remaining salt. Blend until thick and creamy

- You can adjust seasonings to suit your taste.

- You can serve with tortilla chips or nachos.

Braised Cabbage

Nutritionists agree that vegetables cooked in a pressure cooker retain more of their nutrients. Plus, vegetables are more flavorful. Broccoli is the most commonly used, but in this recipe, you'll learn about another vegetable that you can cook in a pressure cooker.

Ingredients

- 1 medium-sized cabbage, roughly 3 pounds (sliced into 8 wedges)

- 1 tbsp. sesame seed oil

- 1 medium-sized carrot (grated, might yield about ¾ cup)

- 1 ¼ cups water

- Another 2 tsps. water

- ¼ cup apple cider vinegar

- ½ tsp. red pepper flakes

- ½ tsp. cayenne powder

- 1 tsp. raw demerara sugar

- 2 tsps. cornstarch

How to Prepare

- Preheat pressure cooker, set to brown/sauté mode.

- In a saucepan, heat sesame oil, and brown the cabbage wedges on each side.

- Add 1 ¼ cups of water to the pressure cooker, sugar, apple cider vinegar, hot pepper flakes, and cayenne pepper. Stir gently. Add the browned cabbage wedges and top with the grated carrots.

- Close lid and cook for about 5 minutes, setting to high. After 5 minutes, open lid with *Normal Pressure Release* (twist valve on the lid to open). Remove the lid.

- Arrange the cabbage wedges on a serving platter. Reheat the cooking liquid (brown/sauté mode), and bring to a boil. In a mixing bowl, make a slurry with cornstarch and 2 tsps. water, and pour into the pressure cooker.

- Boil the cooking liquid until it starts to thicken and pour over to the cabbage wedges just before serving.

Slow-Cooked Beans

This is a flavorful side dish, though the process may be quite long, but your efforts will all be worth it once you're done cooking. This is best paired with your favorite old-fashioned burger.

Ingredients

- 1 pound Great Northern beans (soaked overnight)

- 2 medium yellow onions (diced, may yield 2 cups)

- 1 large carrot (diced, may yield ¾ cup)

- 2 tbsps. vegetable oil (or olive oil)

- 1/3 cup tomato paste

- 3 tbsps. blackstrap molasses

- 1 ½ tsps. Dijon mustard

- 1 ½ cups apple cider vinegar

- 1 tsp. kosher salt

- ¼ tsp. freshly ground black pepper

- 4 cloves garlic (minced)

- 2 tsps. fresh thyme leaves

How to Prepare

- In a saucepan, place the soaked beans. Cover beans with 4 cups water. Set to medium-high heat and bring to a boil.

- When it starts to boil, adjust to medium-low heat. Simmer for 1 ½ hours or until beans are tender with creamy consistency. Make sure not to boil them during this time.

- In a separate saucepan set to medium temperature, heat oil, add onions and carrots, and *sweat* (process of gentle heating of vegetables with little oil or butter), for 30 minutes, or until onions appear flimsy. Make sure the heat does not become too high and stir occasionally.

- Now, make the cider sauce. In a mixing bowl, whisk molasses, tomato paste, brown sugar, and mustard until smooth and even.

Gradually add ACV, whisking a second time until you achieve loose paste consistency. Pour the cider in a slow and steady steam, while constantly whisking to make a fluid mixture. Season with salt and pepper. Add in thyme leaves. Mix thoroughly. Set aside.

- Once you're done sweating the carrots and onions, add in garlic, and cook for about 2 minutes more.

- Gently pour in the cider sauce into the pot with the veggies and stir.

- When beans are done, strain and reserve the liquid for later. Add beans to the veggies and ACV sauce.

- Simmer beans in the liquid you set aside for another 30 to 35 minutes, or until the sauce is thickened. If you have more sauce, simmer roughly closer to 30 minutes. To get thicker sauce, simmer for 45 to 60 minutes. Make sure that you stir occasionally to prevent the beans from sticking into the bottom of the pan. Adjust seasoning to your preference.

- You may cool leftovers first before putting in an airtight container. You can put this in the refrigerator and it can remain fresh up a week, but if you put it inside the freezer, you can extend it to 1 month. When you are reheating, add a few tablespoons of water to loosen the sauce as it becomes warm.

Colorful Garden Salad

This could be a great salad to lift you up when you're having a bad day. It's got colors and the taste is good. You can pair this with warm tortilla with butter. It's perfect for lunch on a slow Sunday at home.

Ingredients

Slaw:

- 1 bunch collard greens (thinly sliced)
- 2 red apple (cored, julienned)
- 2 medium-sized carrots (julienned)
- ½ bunch flat-leaf Italian parsley (finely chopped)
- ½ small head of red cabbage (finely shredded)
- ½ cup pomegranate seeds
- 3 green onions (sliced thinly)
- 1/3 cup sesame seeds (toasted)
- Kosher salt
- Black pepper

Dressing:

- ¼ teaspoon Dijon mustard
- ¼ cup tahini
- 1 teaspoon honey
- ¼ cup apple cider vinegar
- A pinch of kosher salt

How to Prepare

- In a large salad bowl, mix together all the ingredients for the slaw.

- For the dressing, whisk mustard, tahini, honey, vinegar, and salt until you get a smooth and creamy consistency. Add water (1 tsp. at a time) if the dressing becomes too thick or clumpy.

- Toss the dressing with the veggie salad. Top with the excess pomegranate seeds on top before serving.

Tomato Chutney with Apple Cider Vinegar

Tomato chutney goes well with anything. If you want something different, try this chutney recipe with your favorite grilled cheese sandwich.

Ingredients

- 1 ¼ pounds tomatoes (chopped, may yield 3 cups)

- ½ cup raisins

- 1 tbsp. pickling spices

- 1 tbsp. olive oil

- 1 large shallot (chopped)

- 2 tbsps. brown sugar

- ½ tsp. salt

- ½ cup apple cider vinegar

How to Prepare

- Combine all the pickling spices in a piece of clean cheesecloth and set aside.

- Using a stainless-steel pan set to medium heat, put olive oil. Add shallot and sauté.

- Add all the remaining ingredients to the pan. Bring to a boil.

- Reduce heat and simmer. Keep it uncovered, while stirring occasionally, for about 20 minutes.

- Adjust seasoning to your preference.

- Continue simmering for another 30 minutes, or until it thickens.

- Remove from heat and let it cool. Discard the pickling spices.

- When completely cooled, transfer to an airtight container. You can store it in the refrigerator for up to one month. You can also store inside the freezer.

Note: It is up to you what pickling spices you want to include. Recommendation: dill seeds, coriander, mustard seeds, bay leaves, allspice, chili, cinnamon, cloves, and ginger.

Barbecue Sauce with Apple Cider Vinegar

Ingredients

- ½ cup apple sauce
- 2 cups ketchup
- 1/3 cup apple cider vinegar
- ½ cup apple cider
- ¼ cup Worcestershire sauce
- ¾ tsp. garlic powder
- ½ tsp. onion powder
- ¼ tsp. freshly-ground pepper
- 2 tsp. Dijon mustard
- 1 tsp. kosher salt

How to Prepare

- In a saucepan, put apple sauce, ketchup, apple cider vinegar, apple cider, Dijon mustard, Worcestershire sauce, garlic powder, onion powder, salt, and pepper.
- Simmer for about 15 minutes over medium heat.
- Let it cool before transferring to a Mason jar or bottle.
- Serve as desired.

Grapefruit Drink with Apple Cider Vinegar

This is perfect for every meal. Rather than drinking soda, this is better.

Ingredients

- 1 ½ cup fresh grapefruit juice
- 2 tsp. honey
- 2 tsp. apple cider vinegar

How to Prepare

- Mix all these ingredients together and enjoy.
- This is also ideal for people who are trying to lose weight. (More on this in another chapter.)

Not Your Ordinary Apple Pie

It's time to make some changes to your favorite traditional apple pie.

Ingredients

- *For cookie crust:* 1 package of oatmeal cookie mix (including all the other ingredients indicated in the pack, needed to make the crust.

- *For caramel sauce:*

  1 stick of unsalted butter

  3 tbsps. flour

  ½ cup sugar

  ½ cup brown sugar

  ¼ cup apple cider vinegar

- *For the cream filling:*

  1 pack softened cream cheese (8-oz package)

  1 cup milk

  1 pack vanilla pudding mix (3.4-oz package)

  ½ tsp. cinnamon

  1 cup thawed cool whip topping

  ¼ cup cider caramel sauce

How to Prepare

- Preheat your oven to 375°F.

- *Prepare the cookie crust:* Make the dough per package instructions. Then, press dough on a 9" greased pie plate. Bake for about 20 minutes, or until cookie has set. Press down the cookie with a spatula or measuring cup. Place on a dish towel inside the refrigerator to cool down.

- *Prepare the caramel sauce:* Melt the butter in a saucepan. And then whisk in the flour until it thickens like paste. Fold in both sugars and apple cider vinegar. Mix thoroughly, until sauce is thick. Get ¼ cup. Set aside.

- *Prepare the creamy filling:* Beat the cream cheese in a mixing bowl for about a minute or until fluffy. Add in milk, cinnamon, pudding mix, cinnamon, and the apple cider caramel sauce you just prepared. Whip until smooth, might take about 2 to 3 minutes. Pour over the oatmeal crust. Even out layer with a spatula. Chill in the refrigerator, roughly 3 to 4 hours max.

- Add cool whip on top, sprinkle some cinnamon, and drizzle some caramel sauce when you serve.

Apple Cider-Pumpkin Butter

Ingredients

- 1 can pumpkin puree

- ½ cup apple cider vinegar

- ¼ cup maple syrup

- 1/3 cup light brown sugar

- 1 ½ tsp. ground cinnamon

- 1 tsp. vanilla

- ¼ tsp. nutmeg

- A pinch of salt

How to Prepare

- In a small saucepan, combine all the ingredients and simmer over medium-low heat for about 20 minutes or until you get a thick consistency.

- Let it cool before storing in an airtight container.

- Put in the refrigerator.

- Spread on toast or over pancakes. You can also serve it as dipping for apples.

Grilled Chicken

Ingredients

- 1 whole chicken (about 4 pounds), cut into 6 to 8 pieces

Brine:

- ¾ cup coarse kosher salt
- 1/3 cup light brown sugar
- Freshly ground black pepper

Basting Liquid:

- ¼ cup canola oil (with extra to be used for the grate)
- ½ cup apple cider vinegar
- 2 tbsps. Worcestershire sauce
- 1 tbsp. hot sauce

How to Prepare

For the brine:

- Combine brown sugar, salt, and 1 gallon cold water in a plastic container.
- Stir to dissolve sugar and salt.
- Place the chicken pieces, cover, and put in the refrigerator for about 4 to 6 hours.

Prepare the basting liquid:

- In a mixing bowl, whisk ½ cup apple cider vinegar, canola oil, Worcestershire, and hot sauce. Set aside.

Grilling:

- Take out the chicken from brine, drain well. Pat dry.
- Sprinkle chicken pieces with pepper.
- Apply oil to the grill grate.

- Align the chicken on the grill, leaving ample space in between each piece.

- Grill for about 1 to 2 minutes on each side.

- Reduce heat or transfer the chicken to a cooler part of the grill.

- Continue cooking, with occasional turning and brushing with basting liquid. Cooking time is roughly 18 to 20 minutes.

- Transfer cooked chicken pieces to serving platter and serve hot.

Baked Chicken

Ingredients

- 6 chicken breasts (boneless, skinless)
- 1 cup apple cider vinegar
- 5 tsp. garlic salt

How to Prepare

- Preheat your oven to 350°F.
- Put chicken breasts in a baking dish. Season with garlic salt, and then pour over apple cider vinegar.
- Bake for about 35 minutes or until chicken is cooked through.

Glazed Pork Chops

Ingredients

- 6 boneless pork chops

- 2 cups apple cider

- ¼ cup apple cider vinegar

- 1 tbsp. vegetable oil

- 1 tbsp. butter

- 3 cloves garlic (minced)

- 1 tsp. rosemary (minced)

- 1 pinch red pepper flakes

How to Prepare

- Rub salt and pepper on the pork chops.

- Set the skillet over medium-high heat and add oil and butter.

- Cook the pork chops in oil and butter until slightly pink in the center on both sides. Remove from heat and transfer to a plate.

- In the same pan, cook garlic until fragrant.

- Add in apple cider vinegar, then the apple cider, and Dijon mustard. Bring to a boil and continue to simmer until sauce is thickens.

- Add the rosemary and red pepper flakes.

- Season with salt and pepper.

- Add the pork chops and lightly warm for about 2 minutes.

Slow Cooker Braised Pork

Ingredients

- 1 pork shoulder roast (boneless)

- 4 cloves of garlic (peeled)

- 2 shallots (sliced)

- 1 rib celery (chopped)

- 1 tbsp. vegetable oil

- 1 bay leaf

- 1 ½ tsps. Dijon mustard

- ½ cup apple cider vinegar

- 2 ½ cups apple cider

- 1 pinch of cayenne pepper

- 2 tbsps. fresh herbs (sage, thyme, Italian parsley), chopped

How to Prepare

- Sprinkle pork with salt and ground black pepper.

- Heat oil on skillet set to high. Sear pork on all sides, about 3 minutes on each side. Transfer to a slow cooker.

- Reduce stove temperature to medium, and add in shallots and celery. Cool until soft.

- Pour apple cider vinegar and simmer, scraping any browned bits at the bottom of the pan. Reduce liquid.

- Put pork in the slow cooker, and then add the shallot mixture. Add apple cider, garlic, and bay leaf. Cover and set slow cooker to low. Cook pork until it is tender but not falling apart, approximately 6 hours. Turn pork over every hour.

- When cooked, remove pork roast and transfer to a plate. Loosely cover with aluminum foil.

- Drain the remaining liquid on the slow cooker into a large saucepan. Set stove to high heat. Discard the bay leaf and other solids.

- Bring the mixture to a boil. When it starts to boil, decrease heat, and continue cooking, while occasionally skimming fat from the top. Reduce liquid to ¼ of its original volume.

- Remove sauce from heat and add in Dijon mustard and cayenne pepper. Slowly whisk the cold butter until thoroughly mixed.

- Sprinkle salt and pepper and the sliced fresh herbs.

- Cut pork shoulder into ¼ thick slices. Serve with the sauce on top.

Quinoa Salad

Ingredients

- 1 cup sweet potatoes (diced, steamed)
- 2 cups romaine lettuce (chopped)
- 1 cup Brussels sprouts (shredded)
- 1 cup chickpeas
- ½ cup quinoa
- ½ cup pecans (chopped)

Dressing:

- 1 tbsp. apple cider vinegar
- ¼ tbsp. apple cider
- 3 tbsps. tahini
- 1 tbsp. lemon juice
- 1 to 2 tsps. fresh sage (chopped)
- ½ tsp. red pepper flakes
- ½ tsp. sea salt
- Fresh pepper (optional)

How to Prepare

- Steam the sweet potatoes for 10 minutes or until tender. Rinse in cool running water and set aside to completely cool.
- In a mixing bowl, put in the romaine, Brussels sprouts, quinoa, chickpeas, pecans, and the sweet potatoes. Set aside.
- In another mixing bowl, make the dressing. Whisk all the ingredients for the dressing. Adjust seasoning with salt and pepper. If you want, you can also add fresh pepper.
- Drizzle the dressing over the quinoa salad and lightly toss.

- Serve immediately or you can chill but not for more than 20 minutes. Garnish with chives and chili flakes.

Roasted Carrots

Ingredients

- 3 lbs. carrots (peeled, sliced – 1 ½-inch long)
- 3 tbsps. olive oil
- 3 tbsps. honey
- 1/ ½ tbsp. apple cider vinegar
- 1 tbsp. fresh thyme leaves
- 2 ½ tbsp. fresh parsley (chopped)
- Salt and pepper

How to Prepare

- Preheat your oven to 400°F.
- Arrange carrot slices in 12-inch baking sheet (rimmed with wax paper). Drizzle with olive oil, season with salt and pepper, and toss. Spread into an even layer.
- Roast in the oven for 20 minutes. Set aside.
- In a mixing bowl, mix honey and apple cider vinegar. Drizzle into the carrots and toss lightly.
- Return the carrots to the oven and roast for another 10 to 20 minutes. Remove from oven, toss, and sprinkle fresh thyme and fresh parsley.
- Serve warm.

4 APPLE CIDER VINEGAR KEEPS YOUR HOME CLEAN

Wouldn't it be good to know that apple cider vinegar is not just for cooking? There are a variety of ways to use ACV as a cleaning agent. With regular use, you can keep both your body healthy and your house clean.

Here are just some of the things you can do with apple cider vinegar to clean any part of the house.

House in General

Mop floors

Add ¼ cup apple cider vinegar into your bucket full of water with detergent. Use this mixture to mop the floor. The floor will be cleaner and will look more polished.

Clean wood furniture

Wood furniture may appear dull because of the wear and tear from regular use. Bring back the shine to your wood furniture pieces. Add a few drops of apple cider vinegar to water. You may also add a few drops of oil. With the use of a clean cloth, use this when cleaning your furniture pieces. Let it stand for about one minute, then wipe the furniture clean with a dry and clean cloth.

Clean windows

Mix a few drops of apple cider vinegar in warm water. You can use spray bottle for this. Simply spray on your glass windows and wipe them dry with a clean cloth.

Get fleas off your pets

Take one part ACV and one part water and rub it in to your dog or cat's fur to eliminate fleas and keep them away.

Reduce odors

Whether you have a smelly dog, a smoker, an aromatic meal, or just want to freshen the house up for your family or for guests, ACV works as a quick air freshener. Mix a tablespoon of apple cider vinegar in a spray bottle. If you have some essential oils you might add a few drops too. Then spray the room that needs freshening up.

Freshen the diaper pail

If you have a baby in the home then you're more than familiar with the lovely aroma of the diaper pail. Dampen a paper towel with ACV and toss it in the diaper pail every time you empty it.

Kitchen

Remove bacteria

Combine 1 part water and 1 part apple cider vinegar to clean your kitchen and keep it free from bacteria. You can use it to clean countertops, stovetop, microwave, and others. You don't need to worry about acidity since you are using a diluted version, so countertops are still protected.

Clean dishes

Adding ACV when washing dishes helps remove stains, especially from coffee cups and wine glasses. Just add about ¼ cup of apple cider vinegar to your dishwasher wash cycle.

Clean the dishwasher

You can also use apple cider vinegar to clean and deodorize your dishwasher.

Add to liquid dishwashing soap

You can also add a few drops of apple cider vinegar into your dish soap aside from putting apple cider vinegar in every cycle of the dishwasher.

Reduce odors in your refrigerator

You can use apple cider vinegar for your refrigerator in three ways: clean, reduce molds and mildew, and reduce unpleasant odors. Apply undiluted apple cider vinegar directly to any area with mold and mildew. To clean and remove odor, combine equal parts of ACV and water in a spray bottle, use as a cleanser.

Clean the coffee maker

You can use apple cider vinegar to remove mold or residue build up in your coffee maker. Simply run through with water and apple cider vinegar (without the beans) to eliminate that stubborn residue.

Clean the microwave

The microwave may be one of the more difficult areas to clean in your kitchen, but also the most susceptible to grime build-up. Simply fill a small bowl with one part ACV to four parts water and place it in the microwave. Set the heat for High and microwave it for five minutes. The mixture will form a steam treatment that will be easy to wipe off.

Freshen the garbage can

Toss a paper towel dampened with apple cider vinegar into the garbage bin every time you change the liner. It will cut down on the smell of garbage every time you open the cabinet under your sink.

Cut grease

Have you ever looked closely at the range hood above your stove? The hood, the stove top, and the control panel are constantly getting splattered with food and grease as you cook. Add ¼ cup ACV to 2 cups of warm water and use it to cut the grease from these surfaces as you wipe them down.

Bathroom

Manage mildew

Rinse your bathtub to clean mildew with ACV. Depending on how severe the case is, you may opt to use ACV on its own or dilute with water. You may add essential oils to keep the bathroom smelling fresh.

Clear clogged drains

Pour ½ cup baking soda down the clogged drain, and then pour in 1 cup apple cider vinegar, and 1 cup hot water. Wait at least 15 minutes before you rinse it down using boiled water.

Living Room

Clean wax drippings

If you are spending some cozy and relaxing evening with your loved ones and you decided to light a few candles, it is highly likely that wax will run over. Wait until wax is brittle to the touch before scraping it off with a spatula. Use diluted apple cider vinegar to completely remove the residue. You may soak a dishcloth with the diluted ACV to rub the wax away.

Clean windows and walls

You can use diluted apple cider vinegar to clean windows and walls, and even painted walls.

Remove water stains from the side/center table

Despite your constant reminders to use coasters, the kids still manage to leave water stains on the side tables. You can use undiluted apple cider vinegar to get rid of them.

Clean carpet stains

To remove odors and carpet stains, combine 1 part apple cider vinegar and 1 part hot water. Shake well. With the use of a spray bottle, directly apply solution into the stains, and then dab using a cloth to remove excess liquid. Leave it to dry.

Laundry Room

Clean the washing machine

Admit it. You rarely take time in cleaning your washing machine. You can use apple cider vinegar for easier maintenance. Add 2 cups ACV (like you are adding detergent to the machine) and let it run without the clothes. You'll be surprised at how clean the machine will be after that.

Keep your laundry odor-free

You can make your laundry odor-free, germ-free, and cleaner by pouring 1 cup of apple cider vinegar with each wash cycle.

Remove yellow stains on clothes

Stains around the collar or the armpit can ruin a good shirt. Remove stains by combining 12 cups of water with 1 cup of apple cider vinegar. Soak the clothes with stains overnight before washing them.

Remove wrinkles from clothes

Use clean spray bottle for this. Add 3 cups of water and 1 cup apple cider vinegar. When ironing the clothes, spray on the wrinkles, directly. Hang them to dry.

Clean the iron

You can also use ACV to clean your iron. Fill the water reservoir with ACV, turn it into steam, and let it sit upright for about 10 minutes. Add water and let it sit on steam for another 10 minutes.

Use it as a Fabric Softener

If you'd prefer to steer clear of chemicals and additives but still want soft laundry, put ½ cup of apple cider vinegar in your washing machine whenever you want to ensure a soft batch of towels or sheets.

Freshen up musty clothes without washing

Off season clothes are often kept in the attic or basement. When you need to take them out to wear, you don't need to go to the dry cleaning or wash anymore. Using a spray bottle, freshen up the clothes with diluted apple cider vinegar and water.

Garden

Remove weeds

Yes, you can also use ACV in the garden! Pour ACV directly onto the areas that are usually "infested" with weeds, and you eliminate them from your flowerbeds.

Fertilize soil

Combine 10 ounces of apple cider vinegar and 10 gallons of water. This mixture makes a great soil fertilizer.

5 APPLE CIDER VINEGAR FOR YOUR SKIN

Apple cider vinegar is one of nature's most versatile gifts to humankind. You've learned how to cook with it and how to use it to keep your house clean. In this chapter you will find out more about its beauty benefits. It is rich in enzymes, minerals, and vitamins that the skin and hair can benefit from. It is best to use the raw and unfiltered version of ACV.

If you are not careful, you might choose commercial soaps and facial cleaners that contain harmful chemicals that could result to dryness and roughness rather than the smoothness that you aimed for. There are many natural products that are available in the market, one of which is apple cider vinegar.

Reduce age spots

Apple cider vinegar has alpha hydroxy acids, which help eliminate dead skin cells to reveal a healthier and vibrant new skin.

Aside from being a facial wash, you can also apply ACV to the age spots, directly. Let the areas dry, and then rinse your face with cool water.

Do this twice daily for approximately six weeks.

Restore balance to your skin's pH levels

Aside from removing excess oil from your skin, ACV helps maintain the right balance of your skin's pH levels. It also keeps your skin from becoming too dry or too oily as it also ensures a balance in the production of sebum. You can rinse your face with ACV daily.

Delay the signs of aging

Rinse your face with diluted ACV and you minimize the appearance of the early signs of aging, like fine lines and wrinkles.

Another alternative is to soak a cotton cloth in ACV diluted with water and dab on your face. Rinse thoroughly with warm water.

Eliminate toxins

When you wash your face with apple cider vinegar regularly, you eliminate harmful toxins from your skin, thus leaving your face youthful and radiant.

Here are additional benefits of apple cider vinegar for your skin:

Use it to prevent skin breakouts

If you have a constant problem with pimples or acne, apple cider vinegar is all you need. It is a good antiseptic and antibacterial agent that helps prevent skin breakouts by keeping your skin free from oil, dust, and bacteria. It also helps restore and maintain your skin's pH level.

Here's what you can do:

- In a mixing bowl, combine 1 part apple cider vinegar and 2 parts of filtered water.

- Soak a cotton ball into the solution.

- Gently apply directly on the affected areas.

- Let it dry for about 10 minutes before rinsing your face with warm water.

- Do this a few times every day, for at least 3 to 5 days, or until the pimples clear out.

Acne treatment

There are other methods that you can do to use apple cider vinegar to treat acne:

Option #1

- Dab apple cider vinegar to the affected areas using a cotton ball.

- Leave it to completely dry.

- Rinse your face with warm water.

- Gently pat your face to dry.

- Make this a daily routine.

- For sensitive skin, dilute ACV with water.

Option #2

- Get a clean spray bottle.

- Combine 1 part apple cider vinegar and 2 parts of water.

- Spray on the affected areas.

- Leave it to dry for 15 to 20 minutes.

- Rinse with warm water.

- Do this every day.

- Keep the spray bottle inside the refrigerator to get a cooling effect.

Option #3

Open your pores and remove all impurities.

- Boil water.

- Remove from flame.

- Add 2 to 3 tablespoons apple cider vinegar.

- Cover your face with clean face towel.

- Use as steam for the face for 5 minutes.

- Remove the towel.

- Splash your face with cold water.

- Do this every day.

Option #4

Help flush out harmful toxins from your body by preparing an apple cider drink.

- Fill a glass with cold water.

- Pour in 2 tablespoons apple cider vinegar.

- Stir and drink it.

- You may add honey or maple syrup.

- Take note that apple cider vinegar may damage your tooth enamel. It is better to use a straw. You might experience irritation and burning sensation when you drink undiluted ACV.

Use as a face mask

Use baking soda with apple cider vinegar to create a simple exfoliant to kill bacteria and balance the pH level of your skin.

- In a mixing bowl, combine 2 to 3 tablespoons of baking soda with 2 tablespoons apple cider vinegar.

- Mix well.

- Apply as face mask.

- Leave it to dry on your face for 10 to 20 minutes or until your skin becomes tight.

- With cool water, rinse your face.

- Gently pat to dry.

- Apply moisturizer.

- Do this once a week.

- Take note that ACV and baking soda can cause dryness. Make sure you apply moisturizer after every process.

Use as an exfoliant

Honey is an excellent antibacterial agent which helps protect the skin from bacteria that cause acne. It also has moisturizing properties.

- Wash face with lukewarm water and a gentle facial soap.

- Massage the face in circles as you wash it.

- Exfoliate using baking soda.

- Steam the face for about 3 minutes – cover your face with towel and lean over a pot of recently boiled water.

- Take 2 tablespoons raw honey. Gently rub it on your face in small circles. It is done when honey becomes too sticky to pull on the skin.

- Leave it on for 15 minutes.

- Rinse your face clean with lukewarm water.

- Pat the face dry. Do not rub.

- Mix 1 part apple cider vinegar and 1 part water.

- With a cotton ball, dab into the mixture and wipe your face in upward strokes.

- Apply oil-free moisturizer.

- Do this regularly.

Remove skin impurities

Mix aloe vera with apple cider vinegar to remove excess oil and impurities from your skin:

- In a mixing bowl, mix equal parts of apple cider vinegar, aloe vera gel, and water.

- Soak a cotton ball and apply on the affected areas.

- Massage your face in small circular motions.

- Leave it on for 15 to 20 minutes.

- Rinse with lukewarm water.

- Gently pat to dry the face. Do not rub.

- Apply a good moisturizer.

- Repeat regularly.

- If aloe vera is not available, you can replace it with witch hazel, jojoba oil, or coconut oil.

Lemon and apple cider vinegar to remove acne

- In a mixing bowl, mix ½ teaspoon apple cider vinegar and lemon juice.

- With a cotton ball, apply mixture on the affected areas of the face.

- Leave it overnight.

- In the morning, rinse with lukewarm water.

- Do this daily.

- Add a few drops of citrus oil or tea tree oil for added benefits.

As a toner

People with oily skin will benefit from apple cider vinegar, because they can safely use it as astringent. It is an excellent source of alpha hydroxy acids which help increase blood flow to the skin and help minimize pores.

- In a clean bottle (you can also use a spray bottle), add ½ cup apple cider vinegar and ½ cup distilled water.

- You may add a few drops of essential oil, like lavender.

- With a cotton ball, apply mixture on your skin as a toner.

- Leave it on your face for 2 to 3 minutes.

- Rinse with cool water.

- The mixture is safe to use twice a day.

- Shake well before application.

For normal skin, you may use 1 part apple cider vinegar and 2 parts distilled water. For sensitive skin, try adding more water, about 4 parts to 1 part ACV, and do not use often. A patch test is recommended, especially for sensitive skin.

As a sunburn treatment

Excessive exposure to the sun's harmful rays causes sunburn, which can damage your skin. Apple cider vinegar has long been used to treat sunburn. It is a natural astringent and helps soothe the pain of sunburned skin. It speeds up healing, minimizes inflammation, and calms irritation and itching.

- In a mixing bowl, combine equal amounts of apple cider vinegar and cool water. Massage the mixture on sunburned skin. Repeat application several times daily until it completely heals.

- You may also add 1 or 2 cups of apple cider vinegar to your bathtub. Fill it with lukewarm water and soak in for at least 30 minutes. You may use this ACV bath once or twice daily, or as needed.

As a razor bump remedy

When you use razor to remove hair, it is highly likely that you'll have razor bump. Do this for relief:

- Soak cotton ball with undiluted apple cider vinegar. Apply on the affected area.

- If you have severe bumps, apply a light layer of honey first. Let it stand for 5 minutes before rinsing the area.

- Wait until the area is dry before you apply ACV.

Apple cider vinegar has anti-inflammatory properties that help soothe the skin. The acid will help soften the skin.

6 APPLE CIDER VINEGAR FOR YOUR HAIR

You know by now that apple cider vinegar is more than just for cooking. In this chapter you will learn how to use ACV as an inexpensive product to keep your hair and scalp healthy.

Here are 10 reasons why apple cider vinegar is good for your hair:

- It is a natural conditioner. It helps achieve cleaner and shinier hair. Works best if used with baking soda (as shampoo).

- It helps improve the hair's porosity. The ability of your hair to absorb and maintain moisture is referred to as porosity. The acidic property of ACV improves porosity as it effectively seals the hair follicles. Hence, it keeps the moisture in, and your hair healthier.

- It helps prevent tangles. ACV flattens the hair surface, which makes the comb or brush to easily glide through your hair.

- It is a good treatment for hair loss. Apple cider vinegar stimulates hair growth.

- You can use it as shampoo. When apple cider vinegar is mixed with baking soda, the mixture becomes a super-powered hair cleanser.

- It's a good clarifying agent. It effectively removes hair product residue build-up without stripping your hair of natural oils.

- Maintains the normal pH levels of the hair and scalp. Hair's pH is mildly acidic. Ideally, it should be between 4.5 and 5.5, quite close to the pH level of apple cider vinegar. Using ACV as a hair rinse will help you bring back the normal pH level of your hair after shampooing.

- Helps reduce frizz. For people who use baking soda as a DIY treatment for their hair, apple cider vinegar is an excellent follow-up to seal the cuticles, keep the shine, and reduce frizz.

- Ideal treatment for dry and itchy scalp. Apple cider vinegar has antibacterial and antifungal properties.

- Helps prevent split ends. Apple cider vinegar smooths the cuticle of the hair, thus preventing breakages and split ends.

As an anti-dandruff agent

Having dandruff can put you in embarrassing situations. Apple cider vinegar is an antifungal agent that can help eliminate dandruff and prevent it from coming back. It also restores the right pH balance of your scalp and cleans hair follicles and clogged pores.

- Combine 2 tablespoons apple cider vinegar and 2 tablespoons distilled water.

- Add in about 10 to 15 drops tea tree oil.

- Massage the mixture on your scalp for about 5 minutes.

- Leave it on for 5 minutes more.

- Rinse with water and shampoo as usual.

- This is safe to use 2 to 3 times a week.

For healthy and shiny hair

Apple cider vinegar has clarifying properties that help remove shampoo and styling product residue on your hair and scalp. ACV also restores the natural pH level of your scalp.

- Mix ¼ cup apple cider vinegar with 2 cups water.

- Wash and shampoo hair as usual.

- Rinse it out.

- Massage your scalp with this mixture.

- Let it sit for 5 minutes before rinsing your hair.

- Do this once a week.

Treat scalp acne

Scalp acne is a result of clogged hair follicles. The acetic acid in apple cider vinegar helps restore the natural pH level of your scalp. It also helps clear pores, disinfect the skin, heal acne and remove dandruff. It also brings order to tangles, thereby leaving your hair soft and smooth.

- Shampoo and condition hair as usual.

- Combine equal amounts of apple cider vinegar and water.

- Rinse the hair with it.

- Let your hair dry naturally.

- Repeat this treatment once every week for a month.

Maintain the pH balance of sebum and hair

Your scalp produces natural oil, called the sebum, which has a pH level of 4.5 to 5.5. When the right pH level is maintained, it can protect the scalp from fungal and bacterial infection, thus ensuring that you have healthy hair and scalp. However, there are shampoos, hair treatments, and other hair products that can change the natural pH level of the sebum, resulting in damages to the hair follicles and cuticles.

It's simple to use: add apple cider vinegar to the water you use for rinsing your hair. It is safe to the hair and scalp, so you can use it regularly.

- In a bowl (or bottle), mix 1 tablespoon (for short hair) or 2 tablespoons (for longer hair) of ACV with 1 cup water.

- Apply to hair and massage scalp.

- Leave it on for a few minutes.

- Rinse thoroughly.

Rinse hair with apple cider vinegar

You can use this hair rinse one to two times a week. It is ideal to use together with your favorite hair conditioner because it minimizes the tangles in your hair. If you have dry hair, use a lesser amount of apple cider vinegar, but for oily hair, you'll need more ACV to make it work.

Ingredients

- 2 tbsp. apple cider vinegar

- 1 cup of water

How to Prepare

- In a mixing bowl, combine ACV and water. Mix well.

- Wash your hair, shampoo, and condition as usual.

- After rinsing with water, massage hair with the apple cider vinegar rinse you just prepared.

- Rinse hair thoroughly.

Do not be concerned about the smell. As your hair dries the smell of vinegar will dissipate.

Consider using a squeeze or spray bottle so you can evenly apply apple cider vinegar to your hair.

For faster hair growth

Hair loss can be delayed or prevented by stimulating hair growth. It can be achieved by maintaining the normal pH level of the hair and cleaning clogged follicles.

- Mix 2 tablespoons apple cider vinegar and 2 tablespoons coconut oil.

- With a toothbrush, apply the mixture to the scalp to remove dead skin cells. (This is to be done before washing your hair with shampoo.)

- Rinse using equal parts of ACV and water.

Remove head lice

Using apple cider vinegar to remove head lice is a better alternative than the commercially available treatments that might contain some toxic ingredients.

- Before washing your hair, apply coconut oil.

- Cover your head with shower cap.

- Leave it on for 4 hours.

- Mix ½ cup apple cider vinegar and 2 cups water. Use this to rinse off the coconut oil.

- With a fine-toothed comb, run through your hair to remove all the nits or lice eggs.

- You may need to repeat this treatment for a few more days, until all the nits and lice are eliminated.

7 APPLE CIDER VINEGAR FOR THE BODY

People consider apple cider vinegar as a "miracle worker." This type of vinegar is so versatile that it can be used for cooking, for cleaning, as a beauty product, and as a cure-all for almost anything and any part of the body.

Sore throat relief

For people who are suffering from chronic sore throats but don't want to depend too much on cough syrup, apple cider vinegar is a good alternative.

In a glass of warm water add 1 teaspoon ACV, 1 teaspoon cayenne pepper, and 3 teaspoon clover honey. Stir the ingredients together until they are dissolved, and drink.

ACV and honey both have antibacterial properties, while capsaicin in cayenne pepper is a good pain reliever. If certain allergies are what trigger your sore throat, ACV can break up sinus congestion and mucus.

Balance the digestive system

Reduce gas by diluting 1 tablespoon apple cider vinegar in 1 cup water (you can also use tea). Drink this before meals. It also helps ease constipation, because ACV will stimulate the digestive juices to facilitate the breakdown of food.

ACV also alleviates symptoms of heartburn. There are theories suggesting that heartburn results from low acid levels in the stomach. ACV helps increase that.

If you cannot tolerate the taste, try adding a few drops of honey.

Whiten teeth

Apple cider vinegar can be used to remove yellow stains on your teeth. You can simply rub ACV directly, then rinse with water. However, it is important to take note not to do this often because it can damage the tooth enamel.

You can also use it as mouthwash by mixing 1 teaspoon of ACV with 1 cup of water.

Eliminate bad breath

Use ACV as a mouthwash. Mix 1 cup of water with ½ teaspoon apple cider vinegar. Gargle for at least 10 seconds each time before spitting in the sink, until the whole cup has been used.

A relaxing bath

After you've filled your bathtub with water, add ½ to 1 cup ACV, then add Epson salts and a few drops of lavender oil. Soak for about 30 minutes for a rejuvenating bath.

Alleviate the pain of a jellyfish sting

Apply ACV directly to the affected area for help alleviating the symptoms.

Treat a yeast infection

Soak for about 10 minutes in the bathtub filled with water and 1½ cups ACV. This may help ease the symptoms.

Remove warts

Apply ACV directly to a wart using a cotton ball. Secure with an adhesive bandage and leave it overnight.

Reduce body odor

If you have issues with BO you can use ACV to get rid of odor-causing bacteria, as vinegar adjusts the pH level of the skin. Dab a cotton ball with a few drops of **ACV** directly on the area where the odor is strongest.

Reduce foot odor

Smelly feet are a common problem and it can be an unpleasant and embarrassing condition. Apple cider vinegar has potent antimicrobial properties that act as disinfectants, which can eliminate odor-causing bacteria on your feet.

- In a basin, prepare 1 cup of apple cider vinegar.

- Add 4 to 5 cups warm water.

- Soak your feet in the mixture for 10 to 15 minutes.

- Wash your feet with antibacterial soap and warm water.

Feel fuller after eating

There is research showing that the acetic acid in ACV helps you feel more satisfied after eating. In one such study subjects were asked to take ACV while eating bread and the results showed that they had noticeably lower appetite for the bread than the control subjects.

Reduce the itch of bug bites

Dab a few drops of ACV using a cotton ball and apply on the affected area to reduce itchiness.

Counter the effects of poison ivy

Aside from relieving itchiness from bug bites, ACV can also provide relief from itchiness caused by poison ivy and poison oak.

- In a spray bottle, combine equal amounts of apple cider vinegar and water.

- Shake well.

- Directly spray on the affected part.

- You can keep the mixture in the refrigerator for a cooling and soothing effect.

Treat fungus

For athlete's foot or other fungal infections you can directly apply ACV on the affected area. You can also try soaking the affected area in a solution of 1 part ACV and 5 parts water for at least 30 minutes every day.

Relief from sore muscles

Directly rub ACV on sore areas of the body to help relieve tired muscles.

Relieve constipation and gas

To find relief from constipation, add 1 tablespoon ACV to your tea and drink this before every meal. The ACV will trigger the digestive juices necessary for proper digestion.

Help get rid of bruises

Bruises are unattractive. Get rid of the discoloration by applying apple cider vinegar on the area. ACV has anti-inflammatory properties that help lighten the color.

Help improve insulin sensitivity

Studies show that taking apple cider vinegar everyday (at least a teaspoon) helps patients with Type 2 diabetes. Even those without the condition can benefit their blood sugar by taking ACV in this manner.

Can be used as a natural deodorant

In a clean bottle, mix equal parts of water and apple cider vinegar. You can directly apply to your underarms with a cotton ball or with a spray bottle.

Help lower blood pressure

The acetic acid in apple cider vinegar may help lower blood pressure.

Clean sunglasses or eyeglasses

ACV has been proven to make a good cleaner for windows and wineglasses, so, you can also use it to clean your eyeglasses and sunglasses. Simply combine equal parts of apple cider vinegar and water, dip a cloth in the mixture, and wipe your lenses with it. Your glasses will be sparkling clean and streak-free again.

8 LOSE WEIGHT WITH APPLE CIDER VINEGAR

People who have been trying to get fit and lose weight may have tried everything – weight loss pills, fad diets, commercial treatment, and even surgical procedures. Weight loss pills have not yet been proven to make people lose weight fast. Fad diets come ago – some may give positive results, while some can be complete failures.

Pills, fad diets, and other commercial treatments may prove to be effective only for some time, while some do not produce any positive effect at all. Most individuals are not too keen to undergoing surgery just to lose weight.

Apple cider vinegar is a "superfood" that can aid in losing weight, naturally and safely.

The best weight loss technique is to eat nutritional food and to exercise. But for an added bonus, apple cider vinegar will help boost your body's metabolism, thereby letting you burn fat faster and eventually losing excess weight.

Why Apple Cider Vinegar Can Help You Lose Weight

Here are some of the things that apple cider vinegar does for triggering faster weight loss:

- ACV has beta carotene, which can break down and eliminate fat from the body.

- The essential vitamins, minerals, organic acids, and enzymes in ACV may boost metabolism to prevent fat accumulation and quickly burn fat.

- ACV has high properties that help absorb toxins and improve bowel movement, thus, detoxifying your body.

- It has high potassium and fiber content, which help decrease glucose levels in the blood, thus helping control your sugar cravings and prevent binge eating.

- It prevents water retention in the body.

- ACV improves your health in general. It helps regulate cholesterol levels, fight bacteria that cause infections, and improve oxygen flow in the body.

Trigger Weight Loss

Drink this on an empty stomach 30 minutes before eating lunch or dinner. It will help improve your digestion and make you feel satiated, helping you eat less.

- Simply add 1 tbsp. ACV to a glass of warm water. Mix and drink.

- Alternatively, you can add ACV to your fruit or vegetable juice, even tea, but make sure it is not piping hot.

You can enhance the flavor of your drink by adding a variety of ingredients. Here are a few recommendations:

- Honey helps increase your energy levels and helps suppress appetite. It also facilitates the digestive process and boosts your body's metabolism. Add 1 tablespoon to your ACV drink.

- Lemon has pectin which helps prevent hunger pangs. It also aids in flushing out toxins. It also improves the functionality of your vital organs. Add 1 tablespoon lemon juice to the drink.

- Maple syrup is a good alternative if you have allergy to pollen. It enhances digestion and provides additional vitamins and minerals. It is also an excellent antioxidant. Add 1 teaspoon to 1 tablespoon to your ACV drink.

- Cinnamon helps cleanse your colon and digestive system from fat accumulation. It also helps regulate cholesterol levels, by increasing good cholesterol levels and decreasing bad cholesterol. It also helps keep blood sugar at acceptable levels. Add a pinch up to ½ teaspoon to the drink.

- Ginger helps suppress appetite, hence, you feel full longer. It helps improves the functionality of the digestive system and gastrointestinal motility. Add a pinch of ginger powder to your drink for addition

- Cayenne pepper helps curb your appetite, boost your body's metabolism, improves digestion, and helps burn fat faster. Add a pinch up to 1 teaspoon to your drink.

Take note that apple cider vinegar may damage the tooth enamel. It is recommended that you drink with a straw.

Additional Uses of Apple Cider Vinegar for Weight Loss

Aside from the apple cider vinegar drink, here are additional ways to use ACV to lose weight. ACV helps improve the taste of your food, and aids in the digestive process.

Basic Apple Cider Vinegar Salad Dressing

Ingredients

- ½ cup apple cider vinegar

- ½ cup olive oil

- 2 cloves of garlic (finely chopped)

- 2 to 3 tsps. maple syrup

- Salt and pepper

How to Prepare

- In a mixing bowl, whisk together all the ingredients.

- Drizzle on your favorite vegetable salad.

Salad Dressing with Herbs and ACV

Ingredients

- ¼ cup fresh basil, chopped (you can also use oregano or any herb you like)

- ½ cup olive oil

- ½ cup apple cider vinegar

- 2 to 3 tsps. raw honey

- Salt and pepper

How to Prepare

- In a mixing bowl, mix together all the ingredients.

- Add to your favorite greens.

Ginger and Sesame with ACV Dressing

Ingredients

- 1 to 2 tbsps. grated ginger

- 2 cloves of garlic (finely chopped)

- 1 tbsp. sesame seeds

- ¼ cup sesame oil

- 3 tbsps. apple cider vinegar

- 1 tbsp. maple syrup

How to Prepare

- Mix all the ingredients in a mixing bowl.

- Drizzle over your favorite salad greens.

9 APPLE CIDER VINEGAR AS TREATMENT

So far, you have learned the different uses of apple cider vinegar, but there is more to it. Really! This chapter will give you suggestions on how you can use ACV to treat even the common cold.

The common cold

Apple cider vinegar boosts your body's immune system, thus strengthening, and protecting your body against infections, like the common cold.

Acid reflux

It might surprise you to know that acid reflux is the result of having too little acid, rather than having too much. Immediately after you drink water with ACV (8 0z. water with 1 to 2 teaspoons apple cider vinegar), your acid reflux is alleviated. Drink this daily.

Minor scrapes and scratches

For scrapes or scratches that aren't freely bleeding but can still smart, add a teaspoon of ACV to a cup of water and dab the wound with a cotton ball or tissue.

Sore or strep throat

This is unfortunately quite a common ailment for certain susceptible individuals, but you can ease the symptoms with apple cider vinegar. Add 1 to 3 teaspoons ACV to an 8 0z. glass of warm water and gargle.

Sinus infections

Add 2 tablespoons of apple cider vinegar and 1 tablespoon honey to a glass of warm water. The infection may disappear in just a matter of days.

Nasal congestion

Apple cider vinegar has high potassium content and this element helps slow down the production of mucus. Adding to ACV's potency for nasal decongestion is the acetic acid it contains, which prevents the growth of bacteria. Drink this three times a day – most importantly before bed – when suffering nasal congestion: ½ cup warm water mixed with ½ cup ACV and 1 teaspoon honey.

Blood pressure levels

Millions of adults in the United States experience high blood pressure during at least one period in their lives. Studies show that one in three adult Americans are diagnosed with high blood pressure. Taking 2 tablespoons of apple cider vinegar a day may help regulate your blood pressure in as little as one month.

Hiccups

A research showed that chronic hiccups are caused by low stomach acid which slows down the digestion of protein. There is further evidence that shows too much sugary and fatty foods may derail the digestive process by preventing fermentation of food. The most common cause of hiccups is too much eating, though. ACV may help restore the acid balance in your stomach, thereby alleviating spasms experienced by the diaphragm, so you eliminate chronic hiccups.

Swimmer's ear

ACV is a known potent disinfectant. Mix a few drops of apple cider vinegar with water and rubbing alcohol and use as an ear drop. Many people recognize this as one of the best home cures for swimmer's ear.

Hormone imbalances

When you drink ACV before every meal, it will help your body become more efficient in converting proteins from the food you eat into amino acids. These amino acids are essential in many processes to make your body healthy, which includes the synthesis of hormones that regulate functions related to your moods and weight loss. Drinking diluted ACV roughly 30 minutes before meals will help improve your mood, makes you feel relaxed, helps maintain your focus, and promote weight loss.

Insect repellent

You can use apple cider vinegar as a natural skin repellent. Fill half of a large spray bottle (or airtight container), with apple cider vinegar. Add some or all of these herbs: lavender, thyme, sage, mint, and catnip. Then add water to fill up the remaining half. Shake well and let it stand overnight. You can directly spray the solution to your skin to ward off those annoying bugs and insects.

You can also add to 32 oz. apple cider vinegar the following: 2 tbsps. each of dried sage, thyme, rosemary, mint, and lavender. Make sure storage is tightly sealed. Shake well once every day, for 3 weeks. By the end of the third week, strain the liquid and fill spray bottles with ½ ACV and herbs mixture and ½ water. Shake well before spraying on skin.

CONCLUSION

Thank you for taking the time to read this book.

You should now have a good understanding of apple cider vinegar (ACV) — and its uses for cleaning, beauty, cooking, and health.

If you enjoyed this book, please take the time to leave me a review on Amazon. I appreciate your honest feedback, and it really helps me to continue producing high-quality books. Simply go here to leave a review: https://www.amazon.com/dp/B074SB33P7#customerReviews.

And please join my mailing list. You can go here to sign up: https://joannehillyerwrites.wixsite.com/home. You can look forward to bonus content, reader surveys, and announcements about upcoming books.

ABOUT THE AUTHOR

Joanne Hillyer has a lifelong interest in wellness, healthy eating, alternative medicine, and the outdoors. She is especially interested in using easily found tools and ingredients for improving healthy living. Born and raised in the Pacific Northwest, she enjoys the great outdoors, travel, cooking, and walking.

Made in the USA
Middletown, DE
29 March 2019